My Mediterranean Lunch & Dinner

A Full Recipe Collection of Mediterranean Main Courses & Salads

Carmen Berlanti

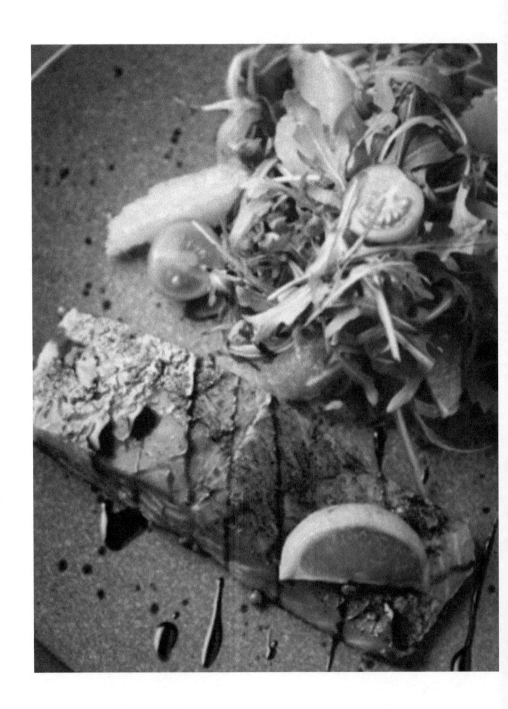

By reading this document, the reader agrees that under no circumstances is the author responsible for any losses, direct or indirect, which are incurred as a result of the use of information contained within this document, including, but not limited to, — errors, omissions, or inaccuracies.

Table of Contents

Crispy Italian Chicken

Difficulty Level: 2/5

Preparation time: 10 minutes

Cooking time: 20 minutes

Servings: 4

Ingredients:

4 chicken legs

1 tsp. dried basil

1 tsp. dried oregano

Salt and pepper

3 tbsps. olive oil

1 tbsp. balsamic vinegar

Directions:

Season the chicken with salt, pepper, basil, and oregano.

Using a skillet, add oil and heat. Add the chicken in the hot oil.

Let each side cook for 5 minutes until golden then cover the skillet with a lid.

Adjust your heat to medium and cook for 10 minutes on one side then flip the chicken repeatedly, cooking for another 10 minutes until crispy.

Serve the chicken and enjoy.

Nutrition:

Calories: 262

Fat: 13.9 g

Sat. fat: 4 g

Fiber: 0 g

Carbohydrates: 0.3 g

Sugar: 0 g

Protein: 32.6 g

Sodium: 405 mg

Chili Oregano Baked Cheese

Difficulty Level: 2/5

Preparation time: 5 minutes

Cooking time: 25 minutes

Servings: 4

Ingredients:

8 oz. or 226.7g feta cheese

4 oz. or 113g mozzarella, crumbled

1 sliced chili pepper

1 tsp. dried oregano

2 tbsps. olive oil

Directions:

Place the feta cheese in a small deep-dish baking pan.

Top with the mozzarella then season with pepper slices and oregano.

cover your pan with lid. Cook in the preheated oven at 350 F/176 C for 20 minutes.

Serve the cheese and enjoy it.

Nutrition:

Calories 292

Fat 24.2 g

Sat. fat 7 g

Fiber 2 g

Carbohydrates 5.7 g

Sugar 3 g

Protein 16.2 g

Sodium 287 mg

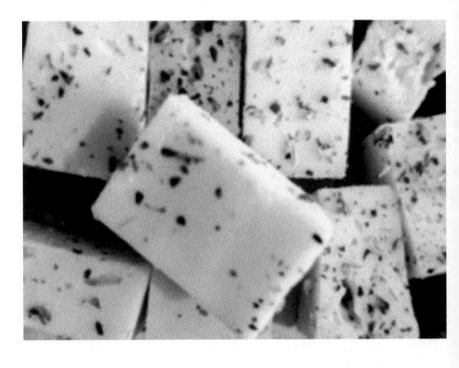

Sea Bass in a Pocket

Difficulty Level: 2/5

Preparation time: 5 minutes

Cooking time: 25 minutes

Servings: 4

Ingredients:

4 sea bass fillets

4 sliced garlic cloves

1 sliced celery stalk

1 sliced zucchini

1 c. halved cherry tomatoes halved

1 shallot, sliced

1 tsp. dried oregano

Salt and pepper

Directions:

Mix the garlic, celery, zucchini, tomatoes, shallot, and oregano in a bowl. Add salt and pepper to taste.

Take 4 sheets of baking paper and arrange them on your working surface.

Spoon the vegetable mixture in the center of each sheet.

Top with a fish fillet then wrap the paper well so it resembles a pocket.

Place the wrapped fish in a baking tray and cook in the preheated oven at 350 F/176 C for 15 minutes. Serve the fish warm and fresh.

Nutrition:

Calories 149

Fat 2.8 g

Sat. fat 0.7 g

Fiber 0 g

Carbohydrates 5.2 g

Sugar 0 g

Protein 25.2 g

Sodium 87 mg

Tomato Roasted Feta

Difficulty Level: 2/5

Preparation time: 10 minutes

Cooking time: 15 minutes

Servings: 4

Ingredients:

8 oz. or 230 g feta cheese

2 peeled tomatoes, diced

2 garlic cloves, chopped

1 c. tomato juice

1 thyme sprig

1 oregano sprig

Directions:

Mix the tomatoes, garlic, tomato juice, thyme, and oregano in a small deep-dish baking pan.

Place the feta cheese on top and cover with aluminum foil.

Cook in the preheated oven at 350 F/176 C for 10-15 minutes.

Serve hot.

Nutrition:

Calories 173

Fat 12.2 g

Sat fat 6 g

Fiber 2 g

Carbohydrates 7.8 g

Sugars 5 g

Protein 9.2 g

Sodium 934 mg

Shrimp, Avocado and Feta Wrap

Difficulty Level: 2/5

Preparation time: 15 minutes

Cooking time: 10 minutes

Servings: 2

Ingredients:

3 oz. or 85g chopped shrimps, cooked

1 tbsp. lime juice

2 tbsps. crumbled feta cheese

¼ c. diced avocado

1 whole-wheat tortilla

¼ c. diced tomato

1 sliced scallion

Directions:

On a non-stick skillet add shrimps and cook for 5 minutes or until nice pink color

Add feta cheese on the tortilla's one side

Top cheese with the rest ingredients. Add the shrimp on the top so they will be in the middle of the wrap when you roll it.

Add lime juice to give it the tangy zing to the wrap.

Then roll the wrap tightly, but make sure that the ingredients don't fall off.

Then cut the wrap in two halves and serve it.

Nutrition:

Calories 371

Fat 14 g

Sat fat 4 g

Fiber 6 g

Carbohydrates 34 g

Sugars 6 g

Protein 29 g

Sodium 34 mg

Broiled Tilapia Parmesan

Difficulty Level: 2/5

Preparation time: 15 minutes

Cooking time: 15 minutes

Servings: 8

Ingredients:

½ c. Parmesan cheese

¼ c. butter, soft

3 tbsps. mayonnaise

2 tbsps. fresh lemon juice

¼ tsp. dried basil

¼ tsp. ground black pepper

1/8 tsp. onion powder

1/8 tsp. celery salt

2 lbs. or 900 g Tilapia fillets

Directions:

Preheat the grill on your oven. Cover a drip tray or grill pan with aluminum foil.

Combine parmesan, butter, mayonnaise, and lemon juice in a small bowl. Apply a seasoning of onion powder, pepper, dried basil, and celery salt mix well and set aside.

Set the fillets in a single layer on the prepared dish. Grill a few centimeters from the heat for 2 to 3 minutes, turn the fillets and grill for a few minutes.

Remove from oven and cover with Parmesan cheese mixture on top.

Grill for another 2 minutes or until the garnish is golden brown and fish flakes easily with a fork. Be careful not to overcook the fish.

Serve and enjoy!

Nutrition:

Calories 224

Fat 12.8 g

Sat fat 3 g

Fiber 0.2 g

Carbohydrates 0.8 g

Sugars 0 g

Protein 25.4 g

Sodium 220mg

Italian Herb Grilled Chicken

Difficulty Level: 2/5

Preparation time: 10 minutes

Cooking time: 20 minutes

Servings: 4

Ingredients:

½ c. lemon juice

½ c. extra-virgin olive oil

3 tbsps. minced garlic

2 tsps. dried oregano

1 tsp. red pepper flakes

1 tsp. salt

2 lbs. or 900 g boneless chicken breasts, skinless

Directions:

In a medium bowl, combine garlic, lemon juice, olive oil, oregano, red pepper flakes, and salt.

Divide chicken breast horizontally to get 2 thin pieces. Repeat this process with the rest chicken breasts.

Set the chicken in the bowl with the marinade and let sit for at least 10 minutes before cooking.

Place the skillet on a high heat and add oil.

Cook each side of the breasts for 4 minutes.

Serve warm.

Nutrition:

Calories 479

Fat 32 g

Sat fat 5 g

Fiber 1 g

Carbohydrates 5 g

Sugars 1 g

Protein 47 g

Sodium 943 mg

Pasta with Creamy Tomato Sauce

Difficulty Level: 3/5

Preparation time: 10 minutes

Cooking time: 10 minutes

Servings: 4

Ingredients:

16 ounces linguine

2 cups chopped onion

1 cup chopped carrot

½ cup dry white wine

½ cup raw unsalted cashew pieces

¼ to ½ cup of water

2 (14.5-ounce) cans diced tomatoes

4 garlic cloves, peeled

24 large basil leaves, 12 left whole and 12 cut into thin ribbons

1 teaspoon of sea salt

¼ teaspoon freshly ground black pepper

Directions:

Bring a large pot of water to a boil over high heat and cook the pasta until al dente according to the directions on the package. Drain.

Meanwhile, in a large skillet, combine the onion, carrot, and wine. (If you're not using a high-speed blender, add the cashews now as well.) Sauté the vegetables over medium heat for 5 minutes, stirring often. As you go, add the water, as needed, to prevent sticking.

.Add the tomatoes and their juices. Cook, often stirring, for another 5 minutes.

Transfer the mixture to a high-speed blender. Add the garlic, whole basil leaves, cashews, salt, and pepper. Blend until very smooth.

Serve generous portions of the sauce over the pasta and top with the fresh basil ribbons.

Nutrition:

Calories: 532;

Total Fat: 11g;

Saturated Fat: 2g;

Protein: 17g;

Carbohydrates: 85g;

Fiber: 8g;

Sodium: 503mg;

Greek Tostadas

Difficulty Level: 2/5

Preparation time: 15 minutes

Cooking time: 10 minutes

Servings: 6

Ingredients:

Olive oil cooking spray

6 (6-inch) corn tortillas

7 cups stemmed and finely chopped lacinato or curly kale

2 tablespoons freshly squeezed lemon juice

1 tablespoon extra-virgin olive oil

2 garlic cloves, minced or pressed

¼ teaspoon of sea salt

1 recipe Happy Hummus

2 avocados, peeled, pitted, and chopped

¾ cup finely chopped purple cabbage

2 tomatoes, chopped

2 limes or lemons, quartered (optional)

Directions:

Preheat the oven to 400°F. Spray a rimmed baking sheet with cooking spray.

Arrange the tortillas in a single layer on the prepared sheet. Spray the tops generously with oil and bake for 5 to 10 minutes until lightly browned and crisp. Set aside.

In a large bowl, combine the kale, lemon juice, and olive oil. Using your hands, work the lemon and oil into the kale, squeezing firmly, so that the kale becomes soft and tenderized, as well as a darker shade of green. Stir in the garlic and salt.

To assemble, top the baked tortillas with a generous layer of hummus. Top evenly with the massaged kale, avocado chunks, cabbage, and tomatoes. If desired, serve with lime or lemon wedges for squeezing over the top.

Nutrition:

Calories: 474;

Total Fat: 28g;

Saturated Fat: 4g;

Protein: 13g;

Carbohydrates: 48g;

Fiber: 13g;

Sodium: 307mg;

Chickpea Medley

Difficulty Level: 1/5

Preparation time: 5 minutes

Cooking time: 0 minutes

Servings: 2

Ingredients:

2 tablespoons tahini

2 tablespoons coconut aminos

1 (15-ounce) can chickpeas or 1½ cups cooked chickpeas, rinsed and drained

1 cup finely chopped lightly packed spinach

1 carrot, peeled and grated

Directions:

In a medium bowl, whisk together the tahini and coconut aminos.

Add the chickpeas, spinach, and carrot to the bowl. Stir well and serve at room temperature. Store leftovers in an airtight container in the refrigerator for up to 1 week.

Nutrition:

Calories: 161;

Total Fat: 6g;

Saturated Fat: 1g;

Protein: 7g;

Carbohydrates: 22g;

Fiber: 6g;

Sodium: 38mg;

Iron: 3mg

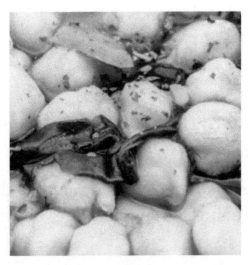

Moroccan Couscous

Difficulty Level: 2/5

Preparation time: 10 minutes

Cooking time: 5 minutes

Servings: 5

Ingredients:

1 cup couscous

1½ cups water

1½ teaspoons grated orange or lemon zest

¾ cup freshly squeezed orange juice

4 or 5 garlic cloves, minced or pressed

2 tablespoons raisins

2 tablespoons pure maple syrup or agave nectar

2¼ teaspoons ground cumin

2¼ teaspoons ground cinnamon

¼ teaspoon paprika

2½ tablespoons minced fresh mint

2 teaspoons freshly squeezed lemon juice

½ teaspoon of sea salt

Directions:

In a medium pot, combine the couscous and water. Add the orange zest and juice, garlic, raisins, maple syrup, cumin, cinnamon, and paprika and stir. Bring the mixture to a boil over medium-high heat.

Remove the couscous from the heat and stir well. Cover with a tight-fitting lid and set aside until all of the liquids are absorbed and the couscous is tender and fluffy. Gently stir in the mint, lemon juice, and salt. Serve warm or cold. Store leftovers in an airtight container in the refrigerator for up to 5 days.

Nutrition:

Calories: 242;

Total Fat: 1g;

Saturated Fat: 0g;

Protein: 7g;

Carbohydrates: 53g;

Fiber: 3g;

Sodium: 244mg;

Iron: 2mg

Alethea's Lemony Asparagus Pasta

Difficulty Level: 2/5

Preparation time: 10 minutes

Cooking time: 20 minutes

Servings: 6

Ingredients:

1 pound spaghetti, linguini, or angel hair pasta

2 crusty bread slices

½ cup plus 1 tablespoon avocado oil, divided

3 cups chopped asparagus (1½-inch pieces)

½ cup vegan "chicken" broth or vegetable broth, divided

6 tablespoons freshly squeezed lemon juice

8 garlic cloves, minced or pressed

3 tablespoons finely chopped fresh curly parsley

1 tablespoon grated lemon zest

1½ teaspoons sea salt

Directions:

Bring a large pot of water to a boil over high heat and cook the pasta until al dente according to the instructions on the package.

Meanwhile, in a medium skillet, crumble the bread into coarse crumbs. Add 1 tablespoon of oil to the pan and stir well to combine over medium heat. Cook for about 5 minutes, stirring often, until the crumbs are golden brown. Remove from the skillet and set aside.

Add the chopped asparagus and ¼ cup of broth in the skillet and cook over medium-high heat until the asparagus is bright green and crisp-tender, about 5 minutes. Transfer the asparagus to a very large bowl.

Add the remaining ½ cup of oil, remaining ¼ cup of broth, lemon juice, garlic, parsley, zest, and salt to the asparagus bowl and stir well.

When the noodles are done, drain well, and add them to the bowl. Gently toss with the asparagus mixture. Just before serving, stir in the toasted bread crumbs. Store leftovers in an airtight container in the refrigerator for up 2 days.

Nutrition:

Calories: 526;

Total Fat: 23g;

Saturated Fat: 3g;

Protein: 13g;

Carbohydrates: 68g;

Fiber: 10g;

Sodium: 1422mg;

Iron: 6mg

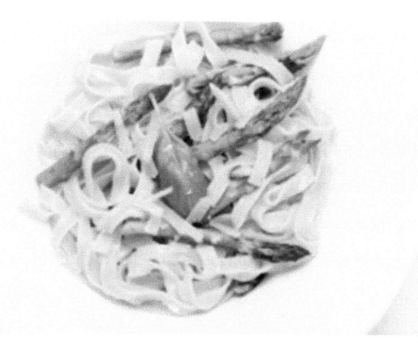

Mediterranean Grilled Shrimp

Difficulty Level: 2/5

Preparation time: 20 minutes

Cooking time: 5 minutes

Servings: 4-7

Ingredients:

2 tablespoons garlic, minced

½ cup lemon juice

3 tablespoons fresh Italian parsley, finely chopped

¼ cup extra-virgin olive oil

1 teaspoon salt

2 pounds jumbo shrimp (21-25), peeled and deveined

Directions:

In a large bowl, mix the garlic, lemon juice, parsley, olive oil, and salt.

Add the shrimp to the bowl and toss to make sure all the pieces are coated with the marinade. Let the shrimp sit for 15 minutes.

Preheat a grill, grill pan, or lightly oiled skillet to high heat. While heating, thread about 5 to 6 pieces of shrimp onto each skewer.

Place the skewers on the grill, grill pan, or skillet and cook for 2 to 3 minutes on each side until cooked through. Serve warm.

Nutrition:

Calories: 402;

Protein: 57g;

Total Carbohydrates: 4g;

Sugars: 1g;

Fiber: 0g;

Total Fat: 18g;

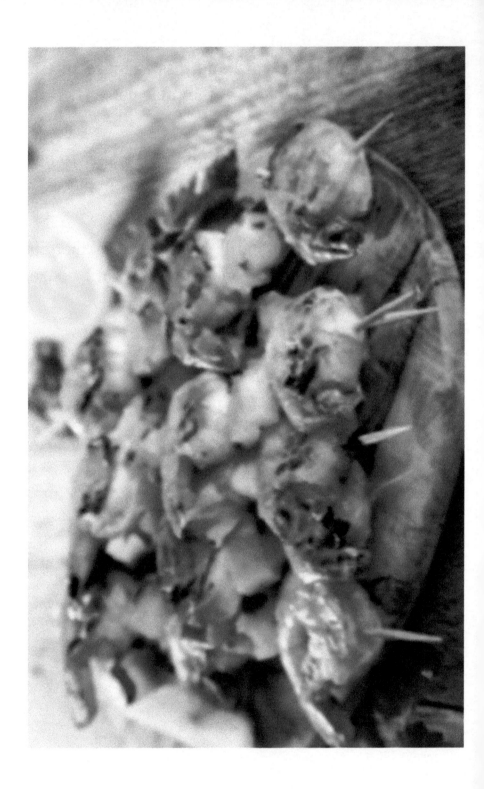

Italian Breaded Shrimp

Difficulty Level: 2/5

Preparation time: 10 minutes

Cooking time: 5 minutes

Servings: 4

Ingredients:

2 large eggs

2 cups seasoned Italian breadcrumbs

1 teaspoon salt

1 cup flour

1 pound large shrimp (21-25), peeled and deveined

Extra-virgin olive oil

Directions:

In a small bowl, beat the eggs with 1 tablespoon water, then transfer to a shallow dish.

Add the breadcrumbs and salt to a separate shallow dish; mix well.

Place the flour into a third shallow dish.

Coat the shrimp in the flour, then egg, and finally the breadcrumbs. Place on a plate and repeat with all of the shrimp.

Preheat a skillet over high heat. Pour in enough olive oil to coat the bottom of the skillet. Cook the shrimp in the hot skillet for 2 to 3 minutes on each side. Take the shrimp out and drain on a paper towel. Serve warm.

Nutrition:

Calories: 714;

Protein: 37g;

Total Carbohydrates: 63g;

Sugars: 4g;

Fiber: 3g;

Total Fat: 34g

Fried Fresh Sardines

Preparation time: 5 minutes

Cooking time: 5 minutes

Servings: 4

Ingredients:

Avocado oil

1½ pounds whole fresh sardines, scales removed

1 teaspoon salt

1 teaspoon freshly ground black pepper

2 cups flour

Directions:

Preheat a deep skillet over medium heat. Pour in enough oil so there is about 1 inch of it in the pan.

Season the fish with the salt and pepper.

Dredge the fish in the flour so it is completely covered.

Slowly drop in 1 fish at a time, making sure not to overcrowd the pan.

Cook for about 3 minutes on each side or just until the fish is golden brown on all sides. Serve warm.

Nutrition:

Calories: 794;

Protein: 48g;

Total Carbohydrates: 44g;

Fiber: 2g;

Total Fat: 47g

White Wine–Sautéed Mussels

Difficulty Level: 2/5

Preparation time: 10 minutes

Cooking time: 10 minutes

Servings: 4

Ingredients:

3 pounds live mussels, cleaned

4 tablespoons (½ stick) salted butter

2 shallots, finely chopped

2 tablespoons garlic, minced

2 cups dry white wine

Directions:

Scrub the mussel shells to make sure they are clean; trim off any that have a beard (hanging string). Put the mussels in a large bowl of water, discarding any that are not tightly closed.

In a large pot over medium heat, cook the butter, shallots, and garlic for 2 minutes.

Add the wine to the pot, and cook for 1 minute.

Add the mussels to the pot, toss with the sauce, and cover with a lid. Let cook for 7 minutes. Discard any mussels that have not opened.

Serve in bowls with the wine broth.

Nutrition:

Calories: 777;

Protein: 82g;

Total Carbohydrates: 29g;

Sugars: 1g;

Total Fat: 27g;

Saturated Fat: 10g

Chicken Shawarma

Difficulty Level: 2/5

Preparation time: 15 minutes

Cooking time: 15 minutes

Servings: 4

Ingredients:

2 pounds boneless and skinless chicken

½ cup lemon juice

½ cup extra-virgin olive oil

3 tablespoons minced garlic

1½ teaspoons salt

½ teaspoon freshly ground black pepper

½ teaspoon ground cardamom

½ teaspoon cinnamon

Hummus and pita bread, for serving (optional)

Directions:

Cut the chicken into ¼-inch strips and put them into a large bowl.

In a separate bowl, whisk together the lemon juice, olive oil, garlic, salt, pepper, cardamom, and cinnamon.

Pour the dressing over the chicken and stir to coat all of the chicken.

Let the chicken sit for about 10 minutes.

Heat a large pan over medium-high heat and cook the chicken pieces for 12 minutes, using tongs to turn the chicken over every few minutes.

Serve with hummus and pita bread, if desired.

Nutrition:

Calories: 477;

Protein: 47g;

Total Carbohydrates: 5g;

Sugars: 1g;

Fiber: 1g;

Total Fat: 32g

Paprika-Spiced Fish

Difficulty Level: 2/5

Preparation time: 5 minutes

Cooking time: 10 minutes

Servings: 4

Ingredients:

4 (5-ounce) sea bass fillets

½ teaspoon salt

1 tablespoon smoked paprika

3 tablespoons unsalted butter

Lemon wedges

Directions:

Season the fish on both sides with the salt. Repeat with the paprika.

Preheat a skillet over high heat. Melt the butter.

Once the butter is melted, add the fish and cook for 4 minutes on each side.

Once the fish is done, move to a serving dish and squeeze lemon over the top.

Nutrition:

Calories: 257;

Protein: 34;

Total Carbohydrates: 1g;

Fiber: 1g;

Total Fat: 13g

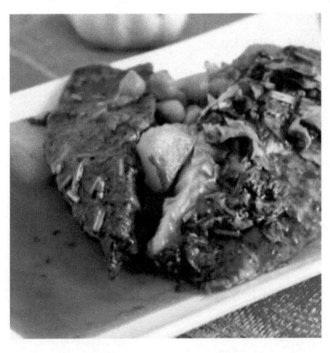

Greek Style Spring Soup

Difficulty Level: 2/5

Preparation Time: 10 minutes

Cooking time: 20 minutes

Servings: 4

Ingredients:

3 cups chicken stock

½ pound chicken breast, shredded

1 tablespoon chives, chopped

1 egg, whisked

½ white onion, diced

1 bell pepper, chopped

1 tablespoon olive oil

¼ cup Arborio rice

½ teaspoon salt

1 tablespoon fresh cilantro, chopped

Directions:

Pour olive oil in the stock pan and preheat it.

Add onion and bell pepper. Roast the vegetables for 3-4 minutes. Stir them from time to time.

After this, add rice and stir well.

Cook the ingredients for 3 minutes over the medium heat.

Then add chicken stock and stir the soup well.

Add salt and bring the soup to boil.

Add shredded chicken breast, cilantro, and chives. Add egg and stir it carefully.

Close the lid and simmer the soup for 5 minutes over the medium heat.

Remove the cooked soup from the heat.

Nutrition:

Calories 176

Fat 5.6 g

Fiber 7.6g

Carbohydrates 23.6 g

Protein 4.6 g

Avgolemono Soup

Difficulty Level: 2/5

Preparation Time: 10 minutes

Cooking time: 20 minutes

Servings: 6

Ingredients:

4 cups chicken stock

1 cup of water

1-pound chicken breast, shredded

1 cup of rice, cooked

3 egg yolks

3 tablespoons lemon juice

1/3 cup fresh parsley, chopped

½ teaspoon salt

¼ teaspoon ground black pepper

Directions:

Pour water and chicken stock in the saucepan and bring to boil.

Then pour one cup of the hot liquid in the food processor.

Add cooked rice, egg yolks, lemon juice, and salt. Blend the mixture until smooth.

After this, transfer the smooth rice mixture into the saucepan with remaining chicken stock liquid.

Add shredded chicken breast, parsley, and ground black pepper.

Boil the soup for 5 minutes more.

Nutrition:

Calories 235

Fat 5.6 g

Fiber 7.6g

Carbohydrates 23.6 g

Protein 4.6 g

Rosemary Minestrone

Difficulty Level: 2/5

Preparation Time: 5 minutes

Cooking time: 25 minutes

Servings: 4

Ingredients:

2 oz celery stalk, chopped

1 russet potato, chopped

½ cup butternut squash, chopped

1 teaspoon fresh rosemary

½ teaspoon salt

½ teaspoon ground black pepper

2 oz Parmesan, grated

1 tablespoon butter

½ zucchini, chopped

¼ cup green beans, chopped

2 oz whole wheat pasta

4 cups chicken stock

½ teaspoon tomato paste

¾ cup red kidney beans, canned, drained

Directions:

In the saucepan combine together celery stalk, potato, butternut squash, rosemary, salt, ground black pepper, butter, and stir well.

Cook the vegetables for 5 minutes over the medium-low heat.

After this, add zucchini, green beans, whole-wheat pasta, chicken stock, and tomato paste.

Add red kidney beans and chicken stock.

Stir the soup well and cook it for 15 minutes over the medium-high heat.

Then add Parmesan and stir minestrone.

Cook it for 2 minutes more.

Ladle minestrone in the serving bowls immediately.

Nutrition:

Calories 234

Fat 6.5

Fiber 10.1

Carbohydrates 39.7

Protein 31.1

Orzo Soup with Kale

Difficulty Level: 2/5

Preparation Time: 10 minutes

Cooking time: 20 minutes

Servings: 4

Ingredients:

1/3 cup orzo pasta

¼ white onion, diced

1 oz celery stalk, chopped

½ teaspoon chili flakes

½ teaspoon salt

1 garlic clove, diced

1 cup kale, chopped

½ cup tomatoes, chopped

1 carrot, chopped

½ teaspoon dried thyme

½ teaspoon dried oregano

5 cups vegetable stock

Directions:

Pour the vegetable stock in the pan and bring it to boil.

Add celery stalk and diced onion.

After this, sprinkle the liquid with chili flakes and salt.

Add diced garlic, tomatoes, carrot, dried thyme, and dried oregano.

Bring the liquid to boil.

Add orzo pasta and cook it for 5 minutes.

After this, add kale and cook the soup for 3 minutes more.

Remove the soup from the heat and leave it to rest with the closed lid for 10 minutes.

Nutrition:

Calories 74

Fat 6.5

Fiber 5.1

Carbohydrates 2.7

Protein 3.1

Braised Swiss Chard with Potatoes

Difficulty Level: 2/5

Preparation time: 5 minutes

Cooking time: 5 minutes

Serving: 4

Ingredients:

1 pound Swiss chard, torn, chopped with stems

2 potatoes, peeled and chopped

¼ tablespoon oregano

1 teaspoon salt

Directions:

Take a pot and add Swiss chard and potatoes to the pot

Pour water to cover all and sprinkle with salt

Close the lid and then press the Pressure cook/Manual button

Cook for 3 minutes on High

Release the steam naturally over 5 minutes

Sprinkle with Italian seasoning or oregano on top

Serve and enjoy!

Nutrition: (Per Serving)

Calories: 246

Fat: 10g

Carbohydrates: 29g

Protein: 12g

Mushroom and Vegetable Penne Pasta

Difficulty Level: 2/5

Preparation Time: 5 minutes

Cooking Time: 8 minutes

Serving: 4

Ingredients:

6 ounces penne pasta

6 ounces shitake mushrooms, chopped

1 small carrot, cut into strips

4 ounces baby spinach, finely chopped

1 teaspoon ginger, grounded

3 tablespoons oil

2 tablespoons soy sauce

6 ounces zucchini, cut into strips

6 ounces leek, finely chopped

½ teaspoon salt

2 garlic cloves, crushed

2 cups of water

Directions:

Heat the oil

Sauté and stir-fry carrot and garlic for 3-4 minutes

Add remaining ingredients and pour in 2 cups water

Cook on High pressure for 4 minutes

Quick-release the pressure

Serve and enjoy!

Nutrition: (Per Serving)

Calories: 429

Fat: 8g

Carbohydrates: 64g

Protein: 25g

Mushroom Spinach Tagliatelle

Difficulty Level: 2/5

Preparation time: 10 minutes

Cooking time: 5 minutes

Serving: 4

Ingredients:

1 pound tagliatelle

¼ cup parmesan cheese, grated

2 garlic cloves, crushed

¼ cup heavy cream

6 ounces mixed mushrooms, frozen

3 tablespoons coconut oil, unsalted

¼ cup feta cheese

1 tablespoon Italian seasoning mix

Directions:

Melt coconut oil on sauté

Stir-fry the garlic for a minute

Stir in feta and mushrooms

Add tagliatelle and 2 cups of water

Cook for 4 minutes on High pressure

Quick-release the pressure

Top with the parmesan

Serve and enjoy!

Nutrition: (Per Serving)

Calories: 298

Fat: 13g

Carbohydrates: 28g

Protein: 14g

Broccoli and Orecchiette Pasta with Feta

Difficulty Level: 2/5

Preparation time: 10 minutes

Cooking time: 14 minutes

Serving: 4

Ingredients:

1 pack (9 ounces) orecchiette

1 tablespoon feta, grated

16 ounces broccoli, roughly chopped

2 garlic cloves

1 teaspoon salt

¼ teaspoon black pepper

3 tablespoons olive oil

Directions:

Add broccoli and orecchiette into your Pressure Pot

Cover with water and close the lid

Cook on High pressure for 10 minutes

Quick-release the pressure

Drain the broccoli and orecchiette

Set them aside and then heat the oil on sauté mode

Stir-fry garlic for 2 minutes

Stir in orecchiette, broccoli, salt and pepper

Cook for 2 minutes more

Once cooked, then press cancel and stir in grated feta

Serve and enjoy!

Nutrition: (Per Serving)

Calories: 350

Fat: 20g

Carbohydrates: 32g

Protein: 15g

Lentil Spread with Parmesan

Difficulty Level: 2/5

Preparation time: 10 minutes

Cooking time: 7 minutes

Servings: 6

Ingredients:

1 pound lentils, cooked

½ teaspoon oregano, ground

2 tablespoons Parmesan cheese

1 cup sweet corn

2 tomatoes, diced

3 tablespoons tomato paste

1 teaspoon salt

½ teaspoon red pepper flakes

¼ cup red wine

1 cup of water

3 tablespoons olive oil

Directions:

Heat oil on sauté

Add tomatoes, tomato paste, ½ cup water

Sprinkle with salt and oregano and stir-fry for 5 minutes

Press cancel and add sweet corn, wine, and lentils

Pour the remaining water and close the lid

Cook on High pressure for 2 minutes

Quick-release the pressure and set aside for 30 minutes

Add Parmesan cheese on top

Serve and enjoy!

Nutrition (Per Serving)

Calories: 356

Fat: 6g

Carbohydrates: 60g

Protein: 19g

Cod on Millet

Difficulty Level: 2/5

Preparation time: 10 minutes

Cooking time: 7 minutes

Serving: 4

Ingredients:

4 cod fillets

1 yellow bell pepper, diced

1 red bell pepper, diced

2 cups chicken broth

1 tablespoon olive oil

1 cup millet

1 cup breadcrumbs

4 tablespoons coconut oil, melted

¼ cup fresh cilantro, minced

1 teaspoon salt

Directions:

Take a pot and combine the millet, red and yellow bell pepper and oil

Cook for 1 minute on Sauté

Then mix the chicken broth

Place a trivet on top

Take a bowl and mix coconut oil, cilantro, lemon zest, crumbs, juice and salt

Spread the breadcrumb mixture evenly on the cod fillet

Place the fish on the trivet, then close the lid

Cook for 6 minutes on High

Quick release the pressure

Serve and enjoy!

Nutrition (Per Serving)

Calories: 352

Fat: 19g

Carbohydrates: 31g

Protein: 14g

Steamed Sea Bass with Turnips

Difficulty Level: 2/5

Preparation time: 10 minutes

Cooking time: 8 minutes

Ingredients:

4 sea bass fillets

4 sprigs thyme

1 white onion, cut into thin rings

2 turnips, chopped

1½ cups of water

1 lemon, sliced

2 pinches salt

1 pinch ground black pepper

2 teaspoons olive oil

Directions:

Add water and set a rack into the pot

Line a parchment paper at the bottom of the steamer basket

Place the lemon slices in a single layer on the rack

Arrange fillets on the top of the lemons, cover with onion and thyme sprigs, then top with turnip

Add olive oil, salt, and pepper to the mixture

Put the steamer basket onto the rack

Close the lid and cook for 8 minutes on low pressure

Quick-release the pressure

Serve over the onion rings and turnips

Enjoy!

Nutrition (Per Serving)

Calories: 226

Fat: 9g

Carbohydrates: 12g

Protein: 26g

Baked Potato and BBQ Lentils

Difficulty Level: 2/5

Preparation time: 5 minutes

Cooking time: 20 minutes

Servings: 4

Ingredients:

2 large-sized potatoes, baked, cut up into 6 wedges

3 cups of water

2 teaspoons molasses

2 teaspoons liquid smoke

1 cup dry brown lentils

1 small onion, chopped up

½ cup organic ketchup

Directions:

Add water, onion, and lentils to the pot

Close the lid and cook on HIGH pressure for 10 minutes

Release the pressure naturally

Add liquid smoke molasses and ketchup to the lentil

Sauté for 5 minutes

Serve over baked potatoes

Enjoy!

Nutrition (Per Serving)

Calories: 140

Fat: 4g

Carbohydrates: 24g

Protein: 5g

Hearty Lamb Bean

Difficulty Level: 2/5

Preparation time: 5 minutes

Cooking time: 25 minutes

Servings: 6

Ingredients:

28 ounces diced tomato, canned

2 cups beef broth

1½ cup mixed beans, soaked for 12 hours and drained

1½ pounds lamb, ground

1 tablespoon paprika

Salt and pepper, to taste

Directions:

Add all ingredients into your Pressure Pot

Stir gently

Close the pot

Cook for 25 minutes on High pressure on the Stew/Meat setting

Release the pressure naturally

Serve and enjoy!

Nutrition (Per Serving)

Calories: 427

Fat: 12.6g

Carbohydrates: 19.4g

Protein: 27.6g

Mediterranean Kale Dish

Difficulty Level: 2/5

Preparation time: 15 minutes

Cooking time: 10 minutes

Ingredients:

12 cups kale, chopped

2 tablespoons lemon juice

1 teaspoon soy sauce

1 tablespoon olive oil

Salt and pepper, as needed

Directions:

Add a steamer insert to your saucepan

Add water and fill it up to the bottom

Cover and bring water to boil on medium-high heat

Add kale into the insert and steam for 7-8 minutes

Add lemon juice, olive oil, soy sauce, salt and pepper in a large bowl

Mix them well

Add the steamed kale to bowl, toss them

Serve and enjoy!

Nutrition (Per Serving)

Calories: 30

Fat: 17g

Carbohydrates: 41g

Protein: 4g

Greek Orzo Salad

Difficulty Level: 2/5

Preparation time: 5 minutes

Cooking time: 10 minutes

Servings: 4

Ingredients:

1 cup orzo pasta, uncooked

6 tablespoons olive oil

1 onion, chopped

½ cup parsley, minced

1 onion, chopped

1½ teaspoons oregano

Directions:

Cook your orzo and drain them

Add to a serving dish

Add 2 teaspoons oil

Take another dish and add onion, remaining oil, oregano, parsley

Then season with salt and pepper

Pour the mixture over the orzo

Let it chill for 24 hours

Serve and enjoy!

Nutrition (Per Serving)

Calories: 327

Fat: 18g

Carbohydrates: 32g

Protein: 10g

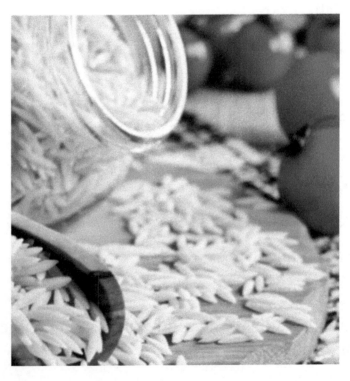

Asparagus Salad

Difficulty Level: 2/5

Preparation time: 10 minutes

Cooking time: 20 minutes

Servings: 4

Ingredients:

1 lemon, juiced

2 salmon fillets

1 tablespoon red wine vinegar

1 tablespoon walnut oil

1 tablespoon Dijon mustard

¼ cup goat Parmesan cheese, shredded

¼ cup fresh mint

¼ cup pine nuts, roasted

¼ teaspoon pepper

2 cups asparagus, shaved

Directions:

Season salmon with salt and keep it on the side

Place a trivet in your Pot

Place salmon over the trivet and close lid, cook on HIGH pressure for 15 minutes

Quick-release pressure

Transfer salmon to a platter and keep it on the side

Add asparagus around the salmon

Take a small bowl and mix lemon juice, walnut oil, champagne vinegar, mustard, and whisk well

Drizzle the dressing over salmon and asparagus

Garnish with pine nuts, pepper, mint and cheddar cheese

Serve and enjoy!

Nutrition (Per Serving)

Calories: 166

Fat: 14g

Carbohydrates: 6g

Protein: 3g

Simple Mushroom Soup

Difficulty Level: 2/5

Preparation time: 10 minutes

Cooking time: 10 minutes

Serving: 4

Ingredients:

1 small onion, diced

8 ounces white button mushroom, chopped

8 ounces Portobello mushrooms

2 cloves garlic, minced

¼ cup white wine vinegar

1 teaspoon fresh thyme

¼ teaspoon pepper

Cashew Cream

1/3 cup raw cashews

½ cup mushroom stock

Directions:

Add onion, mushroom to the Pressure Pot and set your Pressure Pot to Sauté mode

Cook for 8 minutes and stir from time to time

Add garlic and Sauté for 2 minutes more

Add wine and Sauté until evaporated

Add thyme, pepper, salt, mushroom stock, and stir

Lock the lid and cook on HIGH pressure for 5 minutes

Perform quick release

Transfer cashews and water to the blender and blend well

Remove lid and transfer the mix to the blender

Blend until smooth

Server and enjoy it!

Nutrition (Per Serving)

Calories: 193

Fat: 12g

Carbohydrates: 15g

Protein: 7g

Beet and Caper Salad

Difficulty Level: 2/5

Preparation time: 5 minutes

Cooking time: 25 minutes

Servings: 4

Ingredients

4 medium beets

2 tablespoons of rice wine vinegar

For Dressing

Small bunch parsley, stems removed

1 large garlic clove

½ teaspoon salt

Pinch of black pepper

1 tablespoon extra-virgin olive oil

2 tablespoons capers

Directions:

Pour 1 cup of water into your steamer basket and place it on the side

Snip the tops of your beets and wash them well

Put the beets in your steamer basket

Place the steamer basket in your Pressure Pot and lock the lid

Let it cook for about 25 minutes at high pressure

Once done, release the pressure naturally

While it is being cooked, take a small jar and add chopped up parsley and garlic alongside olive oil, salt, pepper and capers

Shake it vigorously to prepare your dressing

Open the lid once the pressure is released and check the beets for doneness using a fork

Take the steamer basket to your sink and run it under cold water

Use your finger to brush off the skin of the beets

Use a plastic cutting board and slice up the beets

Arrange them on a platter and sprinkle some vinegar on top

Nutrition (Per Serving)

Calories: 231

Fat: 20g

Carbohydrates: 11g

Protein: 2g

Couscous with Tuna and Pepperoncini

Difficulty Level: 2/5

Preparation time: 10 minutes

Cooking time: 15 minutes

Servings: 4

Ingredients

1 cup chicken broth or water

¾ teaspoon salt

1¼ cups couscous

⅓ cup fresh parsley, chopped

1 lemon, quartered

2 cans (5 oz each) oil packed tuna

1 pint cherry tomatoes, halved

Extra-virgin olive oil (for serving)

½ cup pepperoncini, sliced

¼ cup capers

Salt, pepper, to taste

Directions:

Add 1 cup chicken broth or water to a small pot and boil it. Turn the heat off, stir in 1¼ cups of couscous, and cover it. Let it boil for 10 minutes.

In the meantime, take another bowl and add 1 pint of halved cherry tomatoes, ½ cup of sliced pepperoncini, ¼ cup capers, ⅓ cup fresh chopped parsley, and oil packed tuna; toss well.

Fluff the couscous with a fork. Season with pepper and salt; drizzle with olive oil.

Top with the mixture of tuna and serve your meal with lemon wedges.

Nutritional info (per serving):

226 calories;

10 g fat;

44 g total carbohydrates;

22 g protein

Lemon Chicken with Asparagus

Difficulty Level: 2/5

Preparation time: 10 minutes

Cooking time: 10 minutes

Servings: 3-4

Ingredients

1 lb. boneless skinless chicken breasts

2 tablespoons honey + 2 tablespoons butter

1/4 cup flour

2 lemons, sliced

1/2 teaspoon salt, pepper to taste

1 teaspoon lemon pepper seasoning

1–2 cups asparagus, chopped

2 tablespoons butter

Directions:

Cut the chicken breast in half horizontally. In a shallow dish, mix 1/4 cup flour and salt and pepper to taste; toss the chicken breast until coated.

To a skillet, add 2 tablespoons of butter and melt over medium heat. Then add the coated chicken breast and cook each side for about 4-5 minutes, sprinkling both sides with lemon pepper.

Once chicken is completely cooked through and is golden brown, transfer it to a plate.

For Asparagus and Lemons:

To the pan, add 1–2 cups chopped asparagus; sauté until bright green for a few minutes.

Remove from the pan and keep it aside. Place the slices of lemon to the bottom of the pan and cook each side until caramelized, for a few minutes without stirring.

Add a bit of butter along with the lemon slices. Take the lemons out of the pan and put them aside.

Serve the chicken with the asparagus and enjoy!

Nutritional info (per serving):

232 calories;

9 g fat;

10.4 g total carbs;

27.5 g protein

Cilantro Lime Chicken

Difficulty Level: 2/5

Preparation time: 10 minutes

Cooking time: 12 minutes

Servings: 4

Ingredients

2 tablespoons olive oil

1/4 teaspoon salt

1.5 lb. boneless chicken breast

1/2 teaspoon ground cumin

1/4 cup lime juice

1/4 cup fresh cilantro

For Avocado Salsa:

1/2 tablespoon red wine vinegar

Salt, to taste

4 avocados, diced

1 garlic clove, minced

1/2 cup fresh cilantro, diced

1/2 teaspoon red pepper flakes

3 tablespoons lime juice

Directions:

Add cilantro, lime juice, 1/2 teaspoon ground cumin, 2 tablespoons olive oil, and salt to a bowl; whisk well.

Add the marinade and chicken breast to a large Ziploc bag; marinate for about 15 minutes.

Preheat the grill to 400°F. Grill the chicken until it's no longer pink, for about 5-7 minutes per side. Remove from the grill.

For avocado salsa: add lime juice, cilantro, 1/2 tablespoon red wine vinegar, 1/2 teaspoon red pepper flakes, 1 minced clove of garlic, salt, and 4 diced avocados to a blender; process well until smooth.

Serve and enjoy!

Nutritional info (per serving):

317 calories;

22 g fat;

11 g total Carbohydrates;

24 g protein

Shrimp And Leek Spaghetti

Difficulty Level: 2/5

Preparation time: 10 minutes

Cooking time: 20 minutes

Servings: 4

Ingredients:

1 lb. peeled, deveined raw shrimp

8 oz. uncooked whole-grain spaghetti

1 tablespoon garlic, chopped

2 cups leek, chopped

1 ½ tablespoons olive oil

¼ cup heavy cream

2 cups frozen baby sweet peas

2 tablespoons dill, chopped

2 teaspoons lemon zest

2 tablespoons lemon juice

½ teaspoon black pepper

¾ teaspoon kosher salt

Directions:

Cook the pasta according to the package instructions. Drain and reserve ½ cup cooking liquid. Cover the pasta.

Pat dry the shrimp and season with pepper and ¼ teaspoon salt.

Heat half of the oil in a skillet over high heat. Add shrimp and cook for 4 minutes, stirring often. Transfer to a plate and cover.

Reduce the heat to medium high. Add garlic, leek, ½ teaspoon salt, and the remaining oil. Cook for 3 minutes, stirring often.

Add cream, peas, lemon zest, lemon juice, and the reserved liquid. Reduce the heat to medium and cook for 3 minutes. Add the shrimp to the skillet and toss well.

Add the pasta evenly to 4 bowls. Add the sauce and the shrimp on top.

Add dill and serve.

Nutritional info (per serving):

446 calories;

13 g fat;

59 g total carbs;

28 g protein

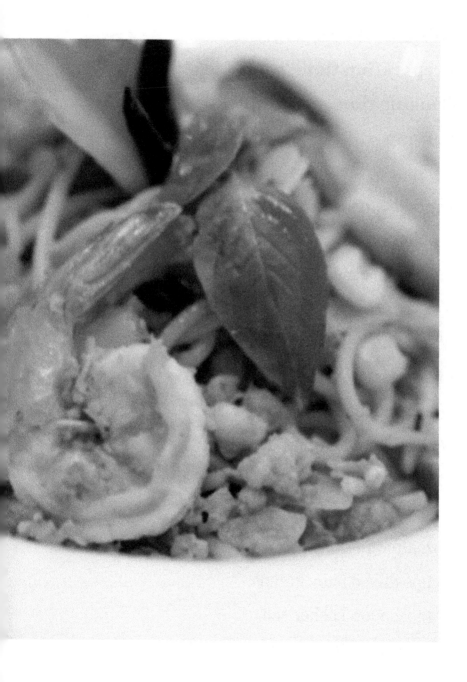

Lamb and Beet Meatballs

Difficulty Level: 2/5

Preparation time: 5 minutes

Cooking time: 20 minutes

Servings: 4

Ingredients

1 tablespoon olive oil

1 (8 oz.) package beets, cooked

6 oz. ground lamb

1/2 cup bulgur, uncooked

1 teaspoon ground cumin

1/2 cup cucumber, grated

1/2 cup sour cream, reduced-fat

2 tablespoons fresh mint, thinly sliced

2 tablespoons fresh lemon juice

1 oz. almond flour

4 cups mixed baby greens

3/4 teaspoon kosher salt

3/4 teaspoon freshly ground black pepper

Directions:

Preheat the oven to 425F.

Add the beets to a food processor and pulse until finely chopped, Then combine the chopped beets with bulgur, lamb, cumin, ½ teaspoon of salt, pepper, and almond flour in a bowl.

Divide the lamb mixture and shape it into 12 meatballs.

Heat the oil in a skillet over medium-high heat, then add into prepared meatballs. Cook until nicely browned on all sides, for about 4 minutes.

Transfer the browned meatballs to the preheated oven and bake until well cooked, about 8 minutes.

Combine the remaining ¼ teaspoon of salt together with cucumber, juice, mint, and sour cream in a bowl, then divide the greens among the serving plates.

Top the greens with the meatballs evenly and serve with the cucumber mixture. Enjoy!

Nutritional info (per serving):

338 calories;

21 g fat;

25 g total carbs;

14 g protein

Chicken Wings Platter

Difficulty Level: 2/5

Preparation time: 10 minutes

Cooking time: 20 minutes

Servings: 4

Ingredients:

2 pounds chicken wings

½ cup tomato sauce

A pinch of salt and black pepper

1 teaspoon smoked paprika

1 tablespoon cilantro, chopped

1 tablespoon chives, chopped

Directions:

In your Pressure Pot, combine the chicken wings with the sauce and the rest of the ingredients, stir, put the lid on and cook on High for 20 minutes.

Release the pressure naturally for 10 minutes, arrange the chicken wings on a platter and serve as an appetizer.

Nutrition:

Calories 203,

Fat 13g,

Fiber 3g,

Carbohydrates 5g,

Protein 8g

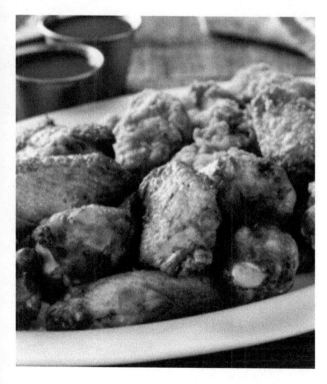

Appetizing Tuna

Difficulty Level: 2/5

Preparation time: 15 min

Cooking time:: - min

Servings: 12

Ingredients:

4 (5 oz.) tuna caned in water, drained

5 hard-boiled eggs, chopped

1/2 cup chopped sweet onion

1 stalk celery, chopped

1 1/2 tablespoons dill pickle relish

2 tsps. honey mustard

3/4 cup mayonnaise

1/2 tsp. celery seed

1/2 tsp. seasoned salt

1/2 tsp. ground black pepper

Directions:

In a large bowl mix together tuna, eggs, onion, and celery.

In a small bowl mix together relish, honey mustard, mayonnaise, celery seed, salt, and pepper.

Combine the mix from the small bowl with the mix from the large bowl, stir gently to coat. Serve at room temperature or let it chill till ready to eat. *Enjoy!*

Nutrition: (Per serving)
 Calories:186kcal;

Fat:13.6g;

Saturated fat:2.4g;

Cholesterol:106mg;

Carbohydrate:2g;

Sugar:1g;

Fiber:0.2g;

Protein:13.6g

Avocado and Tuna

Difficulty Level: 2/5

Preparation time: 20 min

Cooking time: - min

Servings: 4

Ingredients:

1 (12 oz.) tuna caned in water, drained

1 tablespoon mayonnaise

3 green onions, thinly sliced, plus, additional for garnish

1 dash balsamic vinegar

black pepper to taste

1 pinch garlic salt, or to taste

2 ripe avocados, halved and pitted

1/2 red bell pepper, chopped

Directions:

In a bowl mix together tuna, red pepper, green onions, and balsamic vinegar. Season with garlic salt and pepper.

With tuna mixture pack the avocado halves. Before serving garnish with green onions and dash of black pepper. *Enjoy!*

Nutrition: (Per serving)

Calories: 294kcal;

Fat: 18.2g;

Saturated fat: 2.8g;

Cholesterol: 27mg;

Carbohydrate: 11g;

Sugar: 1.9g;

Fiber:7.4g;

Protein:23.9g

Grilled Salmon Kebabs One Way

Difficulty Level: 2/5

Preparation time: 10 min

Cooking time: 10 min

Servings: 4

Ingredients:

2 tsp. sesame seeds

2 tbsp. chopped fresh oregano

1/4 tsp. crushed red pepper flakes

1 tsp. ground cumin

2 lemons, very thinly sliced into rounds

extra-virgin (organic) olive oil spray

1 tsp. kosher salt

1 tsp. kosher salt

Directions:

Spray the greats with oil and the grill on medium heat. Combine sesame seeds, oregano, red pepper flakes, and cumin in a small bowl, mix well. Set aside spice mixture.

Onto 8 pairs of parallel skewers treat salmon and folded lemon slices (beginning and ending with salmon), to make 8 kebabs total. Spray the salmon lightly with olive oil and season with salt and reserved spice mixture.

Grill the salmon, turning occasionally, till the salmon is opaque throughout, around 8 – 10 minutes. *Enjoy!*

Nutrition: (Per serving)

Calories:267kcal;

Fat: 11g;

Saturated fat: 2.1g;

Cholesterol: 94mg;

Carbohydrate: 7g;

Sugar: 0g;

Fiber: 3g;

Protein: 35g

Grilled Cedar Plank Salmon

Difficulty Level: 2/5

Preparation time: 10 min

Cooking time: 20 min

Servings: 4

Ingredients:

1 untreated cedar plank

1 (1 1/4 lbs.) boneless wild salmon fillet

1 lemon, halved

1 tsp. dried oregano

3/4 tsp. kosher salt

1/8 tsp. black pepper

few sprigs of fresh oregano and thyme (optional)

1 cup grape tomatoes, halved

1 tsp. extra-virgin olive oil

1 tsp. red wine vinegar

1/4 cup sliced red onion

1/4 cup Kalamata olives, quartered in long strips

1/8 tsp. kosher salt

black pepper, to taste

fresh oregano for garnish

Directions:

Place the cedar plank in water for 1 hour to soak.

Slice into thin slices 1/2 of the lemon. Use the remaining juice from 1/2 of the lemon to season salmon, and also add oregano, salt, and pepper. Cover and refrigerate till ready to grill.

Combine in a medium bowl tomatoes, olive oil, vinegar, red onion, olives, salt, and pepper.

Place on the plank, skin side down, salmon and fresh herbs. Top that whit lemon slices.

Leaving the right burners off (so you have indirect heat) heat the grill to medium-high heat. Close the grill cover and allow the grill to get hot.

Transfer the planked salmon on direct heat side for 3 – 4 minutes, till the plank start to smoke and become a little charred on the bottom and edges (keep a spray bottle with water by your side in case the edges of plank ignite, check occasionally to make sure this don't happen).

After the 3 – 4 minutes have passed, move the planked salmon to the indirect heat side, close the grill cover, and grill for another 12 – 15 minutes based on the thickness, or till the salmon is cooked throughout in the thickest part (use a fork to take a peak)

When the salmon is cooked, cover it with tomato mix and serve. *Enjoy!*

Nutrition: (Per serving)

Calories:251kcal;

Fat:11g;

Saturated fat:1.6g;

Cholesterol:78mg;

Carbohydrate:8g;

Sugar:0g;

Fiber:2g;

Protein:30g

Arugula Salmon Salad

Difficulty Level: 2/5

Preparation time: 10 min

Cooking time: 10 min

Servings: 1

Ingredients:

1 1/2 cups baby arugula

4 oz. sockeye wild salmon, skin removed

1 tsp. capers, drained

2 tsp. red wine vinegar

1 tsp. extra-virgin olive oil

1 tbsp. (.25 oz.) shaved Parmesan cheese

salt and fresh pepper to taste

Directions:

With a little salt and pepper season the wild salmon, and cook for around 10 minutes, either broiled, on the grill, or in a pan lightly sprayed with olive oil. Put arugula on a dish, sprinkle with salt and pepper and cover with salmon and capers. Drizzle vinegar and olive oil on top and finish with fresh shaved Parmesan cheese. *Enjoy!*

Nutrition: (Per serving)

Calories:288kcal;

Fat:16.1g;

Saturated fat:3.1g;

Cholesterol:66.4mg;

Carbohydrate:11g;

Sugar:2g;

Fiber:3g;

Protein:26g

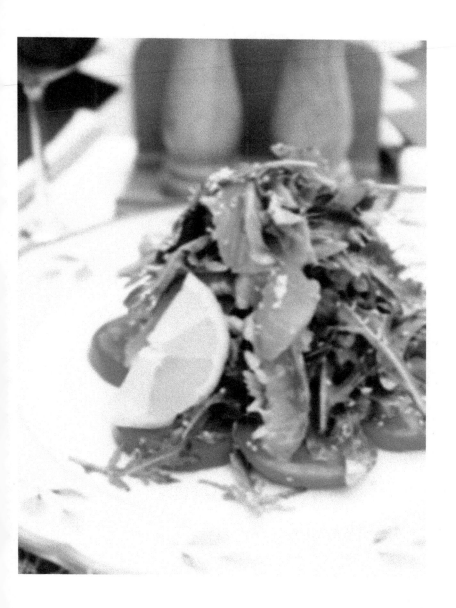

Tilapia With Peppers And Olives

Difficulty Level: 2/5

Preparation time: 10 min

Cooking time: 10 min

Servings: 4

Ingredients:

2 tbsp. extra-virgin olive oil

4 (6-oz.) tilapia fillets

1 onion, thinly sliced

1 onion, thinly sliced

2 red bell peppers, thinly sliced

1/2 cup pitted green olives

1/2 cup fresh flat-leaf parsley, chopped

2 tbsp. fresh lime juice

Directions:

Over medium-high heat in a large non-stick skillet heat 1 tablespoon of olive oil.

With 1/4 teaspoon, each, salt and pepper season the tilapia and cook till opaque throughout, 4 – 5 minutes per side.

In the meantime, over medium-high heat in a second large skillet heat the remaining 1 tablespoon of olive oil.

Stirring often, cook the onion and peppers, till tender, 8 – 10 minutes.

Stir in parsley, olives, lime juice, and 1/4 teaspoon each salt and pepper into the vegetables. Serve with the tilapia. *Enjoy!*

Nutrition: (Per serving)

Calories:276kcal;

Fat:13g;

Saturated fat:3g;

Cholesterol:73mg;

Carbohydrate:8g;

Sugar:3g;

Fiber:3g;

Protein:35g

Cilantro Tilapia

Difficulty Level: 2/5

Preparation time: 5 min

Cooking time: 12 min

Servings: 4

Ingredients:

3 tbsp. extra-virgin olive oil

4 (4 oz.) tilapia fillets, fresh

2 tbsp. garlic salt

2 tbsp. Cajun seasoning

black pepper, to taste

1 bunch cilantro

Directions:

Preheat the oven to 375 degrees Fahrenheit.

Using olive oil coat the bottom of a baking dish.

Arrange tilapia in the pan.

Sprinkle garlic salt, Cajun seasoning, and pepper over tilapia fillets.

Press a few springs of cilantro on top of each tilapia fillet.

Transfer the tilapia into the oven and bake for 8 – 12 minutes. Enjoy alone or with lemon. *Enjoy!*

Tip: Make this into a meal by tossing arugula, baby kale, or other lettuce greens in lemon juice, olive oil, salt and pepper and having as a side salad.

Nutrition: (Per serving)

Calories:200.1kcal;

Fat:12.1g;

Saturated fat:2g;

Cholesterol:56.7mg;

Carbohydrate:0.3g;

Sugar:0.1g;

Fiber:0.2g;

Protein:22.9g

Tilapia Al Ajillo

Difficulty Level: 2/5

Preparation time: 5 min

Cooking time: 15 min

Servings: 4

Ingredients:

1 1/2 lbs. tilapia fillet

4 clove garlic, thinly sliced

3 tbsp. extra-virgin olive oil

salt

pepper

1 lemon, for serving

Asparagus

Directions:

Use salt and pepper to season tilapia fillets.

In a skillet heat olive oil over medium heat.

When the olive oil gets hot place tilapia fillets, and when they start to turn color a bit (after 1 – 2 minutes) add garlic slices.

Cook for another 4 minutes or so, then flip the fillets.

Cook the fillets till cooked through, and the fillets flake easily with a fork (this entirely depends on the thickness of your fillets, so keep a close eye on them).

The garlic should get golden brown color, so if you notice that it is starting to burn, spoon it over the fillets, so it is no more in contact with the pan.

When fillets are cooked squeeze freshly lemon juice over them.

Serve with asparagus and garnish with chopped parsley. *Enjoy!*

Nutrition: (Per serving)

Calories:257kcal;

Fat:13g;

Saturated fat:2g;

Cholesterol:85mg;

Carbohydrate:1g;

Sugar:0g;

Fiber:0g;

Protein:34g

Lightning Source UK Ltd.
Milton Keynes UK
UKHW020720270521
384465UK00005B/135

9 781802 774443